DR. BARBARA'S 7 DAYS CURE FOR DIABETES

Discover Dr. Barbara's proven 7-days diabetes cure: Transform your health with simple step and embrace a vibrant, energetic life

Mauricio Andrea

Table of Contents

COPYRIGHT © 2023

CHAPTER ONE

Understanding Diabetes: Types, Causes, and Symptoms

Diabetes is a chronic metabolic disorder characterized by elevated blood sugar levels over a prolonged period. It occurs due to either insufficient insulin production or the body's inability to effectively use the insulin it produces. Insulin is a hormone produced by the pancreas that helps regulate blood sugar levels. When insulin is lacking or ineffective, blood sugar levels rise, leading to various complications. Understanding the types, causes, and symptoms of diabetes is crucial for effective management and prevention of its complications.

Types of Diabetes:

There are primarily three main types of diabetes: type 1, type 2, and gestational diabetes.

1. **Type 1 Diabetes:** Type 1 diabetes, formerly known as insulin-dependent diabetes or juvenile diabetes, typically develops in children and young adults. It occurs when the immune system mistakenly attacks and destroys insulin-producing beta cells in the pancreas. As a result, the body produces little to no insulin, leading to high blood sugar levels. People with type 1 diabetes require lifelong insulin therapy to manage their blood sugar levels.

2. **Type 2 Diabetes:** Type 2 diabetes, formerly known as non-insulin-dependent diabetes or adult-onset diabetes, is the most common form of diabetes. It usually develops in adults, although it is increasingly seen in children and adolescents due to rising obesity rates. In type 2 diabetes, the body becomes resistant to the effects of insulin, and the pancreas may not produce enough insulin to compensate. Lifestyle factors such as poor diet, lack of physical activity, and obesity contribute significantly to the development of type 2 diabetes.

3. **Gestational Diabetes:** Gestational diabetes occurs during pregnancy and typically resolves after childbirth. It develops when the body cannot produce enough insulin to meet the increased insulin needs during pregnancy. Gestational diabetes increases the risk of complications during pregnancy and childbirth for both the mother and the baby. Women who have had gestational diabetes are at higher risk of developing type 2 diabetes later in life.

Causes of Diabetes:

The exact causes of diabetes vary depending on the type of diabetes.

1. **Type 1 Diabetes:** The exact cause of type 1 diabetes is not fully understood, but it is believed to result from a combination of genetic and environmental factors. Genetic

predisposition plays a significant role, as individuals with certain genetic markers are more likely to develop type 1 diabetes. Environmental triggers, such as viral infections, may also contribute to the development of the condition by triggering an autoimmune response that attacks the insulin-producing cells in the pancreas.

2. **Type 2 Diabetes:** Type 2 diabetes is primarily caused by a combination of genetic and lifestyle factors. Family history and genetics play a significant role, as individuals with a family history of type 2 diabetes are at higher risk of developing the condition themselves. However, lifestyle factors such as poor diet, lack of physical activity, obesity, and stress also play a crucial role in the development of type 2 diabetes. These factors can lead to insulin resistance, where the body's cells become less responsive to insulin, and eventually, to impaired insulin production by the pancreas.

3. **Gestational Diabetes:** Gestational diabetes is caused by hormonal changes and metabolic demands associated with pregnancy. During pregnancy, the placenta produces hormones that can interfere with the body's ability to use insulin effectively, leading to insulin resistance. Women who are overweight or obese before pregnancy, have a family history of diabetes, or belong to certain ethnic groups (such

as African American, Hispanic, or Native American) are at higher risk of developing gestational diabetes.

Symptoms of Diabetes:

The symptoms of diabetes vary depending on the type and severity of the condition. However, common symptoms include:

1. **Frequent Urination (Polyuria):** Excess sugar in the blood draws water from the tissues, leading to increased urine production. People with diabetes may experience frequent urination, especially at night.

2. **Increased Thirst (Polydipsia):** Frequent urination can lead to dehydration, causing increased thirst. People with diabetes may feel constantly thirsty and may drink large amounts of fluids to quench their thirst.

3. **Extreme Hunger (Polyphagia):** Despite eating regularly, people with diabetes may experience extreme hunger due to the body's inability to use glucose effectively for energy. This can lead to overeating and weight gain.

4. **Unexplained Weight Loss:** In type 1 diabetes, the body's inability to produce insulin leads to the breakdown of fat and muscle tissues for energy, resulting in unexplained weight loss. In type 2 diabetes, insulin resistance can also lead to weight loss, especially if the condition is not adequately managed.

5. **Fatigue and Weakness:** High blood sugar levels can interfere with the body's ability to use glucose for energy, leading to fatigue and weakness. People with diabetes may feel tired and lethargic, even after getting enough rest.

6. **Blurred Vision:** High blood sugar levels can cause fluid to be pulled from the lenses of the eyes, leading to blurred vision. If left untreated, diabetes can cause long-term damage to the eyes, leading to vision loss.

7. **Slow Healing of Wounds:** Diabetes can impair the body's ability to heal wounds and infections. High blood sugar levels can damage blood vessels and nerves, leading to poor circulation and reduced sensation in the extremities, making it harder for wounds to heal.

8. **Frequent Infections:** People with diabetes are more susceptible to infections, particularly of the skin, urinary tract, and gums. High blood sugar levels provide an ideal environment for bacteria to thrive, increasing the risk of infections.

In conclusion, diabetes is a complex metabolic disorder characterized by elevated blood sugar levels. Understanding the types, causes, and symptoms of diabetes is essential for early detection, effective management, and prevention of complications. While type 1 diabetes is primarily caused by genetic and autoimmune factors, type 2 diabetes is largely influenced by lifestyle factors such as poor diet and lack of physical activity. Gestational diabetes occurs during pregnancy and resolves after childbirth but increases the risk of developing type 2 diabetes later in life. Recognizing the symptoms of diabetes, such as frequent urination, increased thirst, and unexplained weight loss, is crucial for timely diagnosis and treatment. With proper management, including medication, diet, exercise, and regular monitoring of blood sugar levels, people with diabetes can lead healthy and fulfilling lives while minimizing the risk of complications.

CHAPTER TWO

The Role of Herbs in Diabetes Management: Exploring Natural Solutions

Diabetes is a chronic metabolic disorder characterized by elevated blood sugar levels, which can lead to various complications if not properly managed. While conventional treatments such as insulin therapy and oral medications play a crucial role in diabetes management, there is growing interest in complementary and alternative approaches, including the use of herbs. Herbal remedies have been used for centuries in traditional medicine systems to help regulate blood sugar levels and alleviate symptoms associated with diabetes. In this discussion, we will explore the role of herbs in diabetes management and their potential as natural solutions for this complex condition.

1. Understanding the Mechanisms of Action:

Herbs exert their therapeutic effects on diabetes through various mechanisms of action, including:

- **Improving Insulin Sensitivity:** Some herbs possess insulin-sensitizing properties, helping the body's cells become more responsive to insulin and improving glucose uptake. Examples include bitter melon, fenugreek, cinnamon, and gymnemasylvestre.

- **Stimulating Insulin Production:** Certain herbs have been shown to stimulate insulin production by the pancreas, thereby enhancing the body's ability to regulate blood sugar levels. Herbs such as ginseng, ginger, and berberine are known for their insulinotropic effects.

- **Inhibiting Carbohydrate Absorption:** Some herbs can slow down the absorption of carbohydrates in the digestive tract, reducing postprandial blood sugar spikes. Examples include fenugreek, cinnamon, and gymnemasylvestre.

- **Protecting Pancreatic Beta Cells:** Certain herbs possess antioxidant and anti-inflammatory properties that help protect pancreatic beta cells from damage, preserving their function and insulin-producing capacity.

2. Herbal Remedies for Diabetes Management:

Numerous herbs have shown promise in clinical studies for their potential role in diabetes management. Some of the most commonly studied and used herbs include:

- **Bitter Melon (Momordica charantia):** Bitter melon contains compounds that mimic the action of insulin and help lower blood sugar levels. It also has antioxidant properties that may help protect against diabetic complications.

- **Fenugreek (Trigonella foenum-graecum):** Fenugreek seeds are rich in soluble fiber and saponins, which help lower blood sugar levels by slowing down carbohydrate absorption and improving insulin sensitivity.

- **Cinnamon (Cinnamomum verum):** Cinnamon contains bioactive compounds that have been shown to lower fasting blood sugar levels and improve insulin sensitivity. It may also help reduce cholesterol and triglyceride levels in people with diabetes.

- **Gymnema Sylvestre:**Gymnemasylvestre is known as the "sugar destroyer" due to its ability to reduce sugar cravings and lower blood sugar levels. It works by blocking the taste of sweetness in the mouth and stimulating insulin production.

- **Ginseng:** Ginseng has been used in traditional medicine to improve blood sugar control and increase insulin sensitivity. It may also help reduce inflammation and improve energy levels in people with diabetes.

- **Berberine:** Berberine is a bioactive compound found in several plants, including goldenseal and Oregon grape. It has been shown to lower blood sugar levels by increasing insulin sensitivity and reducing liver glucose production.

3. Incorporating Herbs into Diabetes Management:

When incorporating herbs into diabetes management, it is essential to do so under the guidance of a healthcare professional, especially for individuals already on medication for diabetes. Here are some tips for safely using herbs:

- **Consult with a Healthcare Provider:** Before starting any herbal remedy, consult with a healthcare provider, particularly if you are taking medication for diabetes or other health conditions. Some herbs may interact with medications or have contraindications.

- **Monitor Blood Sugar Levels:** Regularly monitor your blood sugar levels when using herbal remedies to assess their effectiveness and ensure they are not causing any adverse effects.

- **Start Slowly:** Begin with a low dose of the herb and gradually increase it as tolerated. This allows your body to adjust to the herb's effects and minimizes the risk of side effects.

- **Choose High-Quality Products:** Select high-quality herbal products from reputable sources to ensure purity, potency, and safety.

- **Combine with Lifestyle Modifications:** Herbal remedies should complement, not replace, conventional diabetes management strategies such as medication, diet, exercise, and regular monitoring of blood sugar levels.

Conclusion:

In conclusion, herbs play a valuable role in diabetes management by offering natural solutions to help regulate blood sugar levels and improve overall health and well-being. While more research is needed to fully understand the efficacy and safety of herbal remedies for diabetes, many herbs have shown promising results in clinical studies and traditional use. When used judiciously and under the guidance of a healthcare provider, herbs can be valuable additions to a comprehensive diabetes management plan, providing individuals with additional tools to support their health and vitality.

CHAPTER THREE

Getting Started: Preparing Mentally and Physically for the Herbal Cure

Embarking on a journey towards herbal healing requires both mental and physical preparation to ensure success and optimal outcomes. Whether you're considering herbal remedies for a specific health condition or simply seeking to enhance your overall well-being, preparing yourself mentally and physically can help you maximize the benefits of herbal medicine. In this guide, we'll explore key steps to help you get started on your herbal healing journey.

1. Educate Yourself:

Before diving into herbal remedies, take the time to educate yourself about the principles of herbal medicine, different herbs and their properties, and how they can be used for various health concerns. There are plenty of resources available, including books, online courses, and reputable websites, that can provide valuable information on herbal medicine.

2. Set Clear Intentions:

Clarify your goals and intentions for using herbal remedies. Whether you're seeking relief from specific symptoms, aiming to improve your overall health, or exploring alternative treatments for a chronic condition, having clear intentions will guide your herbal healing journey and help you stay focused on your objectives.

3. Consult with a Professional:

It's essential to seek guidance from a qualified herbalist, naturopath, or healthcare provider before starting any herbal treatment regimen, especially if you have pre-existing health conditions or are taking medications. A professional can offer personalized recommendations based on your individual needs, assess potential interactions with medications, and provide guidance on dosage and usage.

4. Assess Your Lifestyle:

Evaluate your current lifestyle habits, including diet, exercise, sleep patterns, stress levels, and overall lifestyle choices. Herbal medicine works best when complemented by a healthy lifestyle, so consider making any necessary adjustments to support your herbal healing journey. Incorporating nutritious foods, regular physical activity, adequate sleep, stress management techniques, and other healthy habits can enhance the effectiveness of herbal remedies.

5. Create a Healing Environment:

Set up a healing environment in your home that supports your herbal healing practices. Create a dedicated space for preparing and storing herbs, such as a kitchen cabinet or shelf. Consider incorporating elements that promote relaxation and well-being, such as plants, candles, calming music, or essential oil diffusers, to enhance the therapeutic experience.

6. Start Slowly:

When integrating herbal remedies into your routine, start slowly and gradually introduce new herbs one at a time. This allows you to monitor your body's response and observe any potential side effects or allergic reactions. Begin with small doses and gradually increase as tolerated, following the recommendations of your healthcare provider or herbalist.

7. Keep a Journal:

Maintain a journal to track your herbal healing journey, including the herbs you're using, dosage, frequency, and any changes you notice in your health and well-being. Recording your experiences can help you identify patterns, track progress, and make informed decisions about which herbs work best for you.

8. Stay Open-Minded:

Approach herbal healing with an open mind and a willingness to explore new possibilities. Keep in mind that herbal medicine is a holistic practice that considers the interconnectedness of the body, mind, and spirit. Be open to trying different herbs, techniques, and approaches to find what resonates best with you and supports your health goals.

9. Practice Patience and Persistence:

Herbal healing is often a gradual process that requires patience and persistence. It may take time to see noticeable improvements in your health, and some herbs may require regular and consistent use to achieve desired results. Trust in the healing power of nature and stay committed to your herbal regimen, adjusting as needed based on your body's response.

10. Trust Your Intuition:

Listen to your body and trust your intuition when it comes to using herbal remedies. Pay attention to how you feel before, during, and after taking herbs, and honor any intuitive insights or sensations that arise. Your body has its wisdom and knows what it needs for healing and balance.

In conclusion, preparing mentally and physically for the herbal cure involves educating yourself, setting clear intentions, consulting with professionals, assessing your lifestyle, creating a healing environment, starting slowly, keeping a journal, staying open-minded, practicing patience and persistence, and trusting your intuition. By taking these steps, you can lay a solid foundation for a successful and fulfilling herbal healing journey that supports your overall health and well-being.

CHAPTER FOUR

Day 1: Introduction to Herbal Remedies for Blood Sugar Control

Welcome to Day 1 of your journey towards exploring herbal remedies for blood sugar control. Today, we'll lay the groundwork by providing you with an introduction to herbal medicine, its role in managing blood sugar levels, and some key herbs that have shown promise in this regard.

Understanding Herbal Medicine:

Herbal medicine, also known as herbalism or phytotherapy, is the practice of using plants and plant extracts for medicinal purposes. It is one of the oldest forms of medicine, with a rich history dating back thousands of years across various cultures and civilizations. Herbal remedies are derived from the leaves, roots, flowers, bark, or seeds of plants and are used to promote health, prevent illness, and alleviate symptoms of various health conditions.

Herbs for Blood Sugar Control:

Several herbs have gained recognition for their potential to help regulate blood sugar levels and support overall metabolic health. While more research is needed to fully understand their mechanisms of action and efficacy, many of these herbs have been used for centuries in traditional medicine systems for their therapeutic properties. Here are some key herbs for blood sugar control:

1. **Bitter Melon (Momordica charantia):** Bitter melon is a tropical vine native to Asia, Africa, and the Caribbean. It contains compounds that mimic the action of insulin, helping to lower blood sugar levels. Bitter melon may also improve insulin sensitivity and reduce insulin resistance.

2. **Fenugreek (Trigonella foenum-graecum):** Fenugreek seeds are rich in soluble fiber and saponins, which help slow down the absorption of carbohydrates and sugars in the digestive tract. This can lead to more stable blood sugar levels after meals.

3. **Cinnamon (Cinnamomum verum):** Cinnamon contains bioactive compounds that may help improve insulin sensitivity and lower fasting blood sugar levels. It may also have antioxidant and anti-inflammatory effects that benefit overall health.

4. **Gymnema Sylvestre:**Gymnemasylvestre, also known as the "sugar destroyer," has been used in Ayurvedic medicine for centuries to help reduce sugar cravings and support healthy blood sugar levels. It may work by blocking the taste of sweetness in the mouth and supporting insulin production.

5. **Ginseng:** Ginseng is a popular adaptogenic herb known for its ability to improve energy levels, reduce stress, and support overall well-being. Some research suggests that ginseng may also help improve blood sugar control and insulin sensitivity.

Next Steps:

As you begin your journey into herbal remedies for blood sugar control, take some time to familiarize yourself with these key herbs and their potential benefits. Consider incorporating them into your diet and daily routine in various forms, such as herbal teas, capsules, tinctures, or culinary preparations.

Keep in mind that herbal medicine works best when used as part of a holistic approach to health, which includes a balanced diet, regular exercise, stress management, and other lifestyle factors. Consult with a qualified healthcare provider or herbalist before starting any new herbal regimen, especially if you have pre-existing health conditions or are taking medications.

Stay tuned for Day 2, where we'll delve deeper into specific herbs and their therapeutic properties for blood sugar control. In the meantime, enjoy exploring the world of herbal medicine and its potential to support your health and well-being.

CHAPTER FIVE

Day 2-6: Daily Herbal Protocols for Managing Diabetes

Welcome to Days 2 through 6 of your journey towards managing diabetes with herbal remedies. Over the next five days, we'll introduce you to a daily herbal protocol designed to support blood sugar control and overall well-being. Each day will focus on specific herbs and their therapeutic properties, along with practical tips for incorporating them into your daily routine. Let's get started!

Day 2: Bitter Melon

Herb: Bitter Melon (Momordica charantia)

Therapeutic Properties: Bitter melon contains compounds that mimic the action of insulin, helping to lower blood sugar levels. It may also improve insulin sensitivity and reduce insulin resistance.

Daily Protocol:

- Start your day with a cup of bitter melon tea. Steep fresh or dried bitter melon slices in hot water for 10-15 minutes. You can sweeten the tea with a small amount of honey or stevia if desired.

- Incorporate bitter melon into your meals by adding it to stir-fries, soups, or salads. Bitter melon is commonly used in

Asian cuisine and pairs well with ingredients like garlic, ginger, and soy sauce.

Day 3: Fenugreek

Herb: Fenugreek (Trigonella foenum-graecum)

Therapeutic Properties: Fenugreek seeds are rich in soluble fiber and saponins, which help slow down the absorption of carbohydrates and sugars in the digestive tract. This can lead to more stable blood sugar levels after meals.

Daily Protocol:

- Start your day with a fenugreek-infused smoothie. Blend together fresh or soaked fenugreek seeds with your favorite fruits and leafy greens for a nutritious and blood sugar-friendly breakfast option.

- Incorporate fenugreek seeds into your cooking by adding them to curries, stews, or baked goods. Fenugreek seeds have a slightly bitter taste that pairs well with savory dishes.

Day 4: Cinnamon

Herb: Cinnamon (Cinnamomum verum)

Therapeutic Properties: Cinnamon contains bioactive compounds that may help improve insulin sensitivity and lower fasting blood sugar levels. It may also have antioxidant and anti-inflammatory effects that benefit overall health.

Daily Protocol:

- Sprinkle cinnamon on your morning oatmeal or yogurt for a delicious and blood sugar-balancing breakfast. Cinnamon adds warmth and sweetness to dishes without the need for added sugars.

- Enjoy a cup of cinnamon tea in the afternoon for a comforting and health-promoting beverage. Simply steep a cinnamon stick in hot water for 10-15 minutes and enjoy.

Day 5: Gymnema Sylvestre

Herb: Gymnema Sylvestre

Therapeutic Properties: Gymnemasylvestre, also known as the "sugar destroyer," has been used in Ayurvedic medicine for centuries to help reduce sugar cravings and support healthy blood sugar levels. It may work by blocking the taste of sweetness in the mouth and supporting insulin production.

Daily Protocol:

- Take gymnemasylvestre capsules or tincture as directed by your healthcare provider or herbalist. This herb is often taken before meals to help reduce sugar cravings and support blood sugar control.

- Chew on gymnemasylvestre leaves or drink gymnema tea throughout the day to help curb sugar cravings and promote a balanced appetite.

Day 6: Ginseng

Herb: Ginseng

Therapeutic Properties: Ginseng is a popular adaptogenic herb known for its ability to improve energy levels, reduce stress, and support overall well-being. Some research suggests that ginseng may also help improve blood sugar control and insulin sensitivity.

Daily Protocol:

- Enjoy a cup of ginseng tea in the morning or afternoon for a natural energy boost and support for blood sugar control. Ginseng tea can be made by steeping ginseng slices or tea bags in hot water for 5-10 minutes.

- Take ginseng supplements as directed by your healthcare provider or herbalist. Ginseng supplements are available in various forms, including capsules, powders, and extracts.

Conclusion:

By following this daily herbal protocol for managing diabetes, you can harness the therapeutic properties of key herbs to support blood sugar control and overall well-being. Remember to consult with a qualified healthcare provider or herbalist before starting any new herbal regimen, especially if you have pre-existing health conditions or are taking medications. Stay tuned for more insights and tips on herbal remedies for diabetes management.

CHAPTER SIX

Day 7: Culmination and Reflection on the 7-Day Herbal Cure

Congratulations on completing the 7-day herbal cure journey for managing diabetes! Today, we'll take some time to reflect on your experience, celebrate your achievements, and explore ways to continue incorporating herbal remedies into your daily life for long-term health and well-being.

Reflection Questions:

1. **What were your observations and experiences during the 7-day herbal cure journey?** Take a moment to reflect on how you felt physically, mentally, and emotionally throughout the past week. Did you notice any changes in your energy levels, mood, or blood sugar levels? What were the highlights of your herbal remedy experience?

2. **Which herbs and protocols resonated most with you?** Consider which herbs and daily protocols you found most enjoyable and effective during the 7-day herbal cure. Did you discover any new favorite herbs or recipes that you plan to continue incorporating into your routine?

3. **What challenges did you encounter, and how did you overcome them?** Reflect on any challenges or obstacles you faced during the herbal cure journey, such as sourcing herbs,

adjusting to new flavors, or integrating herbal remedies into your daily routine. How did you navigate these challenges, and what strategies did you find helpful?

4. **How has your perspective on herbal medicine evolved?** Think about how your understanding and perception of herbal medicine have evolved throughout the past week. Has your appreciation for natural remedies grown? Are you more inclined to explore herbal options for other health concerns or incorporate herbs into your daily wellness routine?

Celebrating Achievements:

Take a moment to celebrate your achievements and acknowledge the progress you've made towards supporting your health and well-being with herbal remedies. Whether you noticed improvements in your energy levels, mood, or blood sugar control, every step forward is a testament to your commitment to self-care and holistic healing.

Continuing the Journey:

As you conclude the 7-day herbal cure, consider how you can continue integrating herbal remedies into your daily life for ongoing health maintenance and disease prevention. Here are some ideas to inspire you:

- **Maintain Consistency:** Continue incorporating your favorite herbs and protocols from the past week into your daily routine. Consistency is key to reaping the long-term benefits of herbal medicine.

- **Explore New Herbs:** Keep exploring new herbs and experimenting with different combinations and recipes. The world of herbal medicine is vast and diverse, offering endless possibilities for supporting health and well-being.

- **Stay Informed:** Stay informed about the latest research and developments in herbal medicine. Follow reputable sources, attend workshops or seminars, and connect with herbalists and healthcare providers who specialize in natural medicine.

- **Listen to Your Body:** Pay attention to your body's signals and adjust your herbal regimen as needed. Trust your intuition and honor your body's unique needs and preferences.

- **Seek Professional Guidance:** Continue working with a qualified healthcare provider or herbalist to develop a personalized herbal treatment plan tailored to your individual health goals and concerns.

Conclusion:

The culmination of the 7-day herbal cure marks the beginning of an ongoing journey towards health and well-being through the power of herbal medicine. By reflecting on your experience, celebrating your achievements, and committing to continued exploration and self-care, you can cultivate a deeper connection with nature and harness the healing potential of herbs for a vibrant and fulfilling life. Here's to your health and vitality!

CHAPTER SEVEN

Integrating Herbal Remedies into Your Diabetes Management Plan: Dosage and Safety

Integrating herbal remedies into your diabetes management plan can be a beneficial complement to conventional treatments. However, it's essential to approach herbal medicine with caution and ensure that you use herbs safely and effectively. In this guide, we'll explore dosage considerations and safety precautions for incorporating herbal remedies into your diabetes management plan.

1. Consult with a Healthcare Provider:

Before starting any herbal remedy for diabetes, consult with a qualified healthcare provider who is knowledgeable about herbal medicine. They can provide personalized recommendations based on your individual health status, current medications, and specific needs. Your healthcare provider can also help you determine the appropriate dosage and monitor your progress over time.

2. Start with Low Dosages:

When using herbal remedies, especially if you're new to them, start with low dosages and gradually increase as tolerated. This allows your body to adjust to the herb's effects and reduces the risk of adverse reactions. Pay attention to any signs of discomfort or side effects, and adjust the dosage accordingly.

3. Follow Recommended Dosages:

Always follow the recommended dosages provided by your healthcare provider or the product label. Dosages can vary depending on the herb, its preparation, and individual factors such as age, weight, and overall health. Taking too much of an herb can be harmful and may lead to adverse effects or interactions with medications.

4. Consider Form and Preparation:

Herbal remedies come in various forms, including capsules, tablets, tinctures, teas, and extracts. Each form may have different dosages and absorption rates. Pay attention to the recommended dosage for the specific form of the herb you're using and follow the manufacturer's instructions for preparation and administration.

5. Monitor Blood Sugar Levels:

Regularly monitor your blood sugar levels when using herbal remedies to assess their effectiveness and ensure they're not causing any adverse effects. Keep a record of your blood sugar readings and any changes you notice while using herbal remedies. Report any significant fluctuations to your healthcare provider.

6. Be Aware of Interactions:

Some herbs may interact with medications commonly used to treat diabetes, such as insulin or oral hypoglycemic agents.

Certain herbs can potentiate the effects of these medications, leading to hypoglycemia (low blood sugar). Others may interfere with the metabolism or absorption of medications, reducing their effectiveness. Always inform your healthcare provider about any herbal remedies you're using to avoid potential interactions.

7. Choose High-Quality Products:

Select high-quality herbal products from reputable manufacturers to ensure purity, potency, and safety. Look for products that have been tested for quality and standardized for active ingredients. Avoid purchasing herbs from unreliable sources or products that make unsubstantiated claims about their efficacy.

8. Listen to Your Body:

Pay attention to how your body responds to herbal remedies and trust your intuition. If you experience any adverse effects or discomfort, stop using the herb and consult with your healthcare provider. Likewise, if you notice positive changes in your symptoms or overall well-being, continue with the herbal remedy as recommended.

Conclusion:

Integrating herbal remedies into your diabetes management plan can offer additional support for blood sugar control and overall health. By following dosage considerations and safety precautions, you can use herbal medicine effectively and minimize the risk of adverse effects. Remember to consult with a qualified healthcare provider before starting any new herbal remedy, especially if you have pre-existing health conditions or are taking medications. With proper guidance and monitoring, herbal remedies can be valuable tools in your diabetes management toolbox.

CHAPTER EIGHT

Lifestyle Changes for Long-Term Diabetes Control: Diet, Exercise, and Stress Management

Managing diabetes effectively requires a comprehensive approach that includes not only medication but also lifestyle modifications. Diet, exercise, and stress management play crucial roles in controlling blood sugar levels, improving insulin sensitivity, and reducing the risk of complications associated with diabetes. In this guide, we'll explore practical lifestyle changes you can implement for long-term diabetes control.

1. Diet:

A healthy diet is essential for managing diabetes and maintaining stable blood sugar levels. Here are some dietary recommendations:

- **Focus on Whole Foods:** Emphasize whole, unprocessed foods such as fruits, vegetables, whole grains, lean proteins, and healthy fats. These foods are rich in nutrients and fiber, which can help regulate blood sugar levels and promote overall health.

- **Limit Sugary and Processed Foods:** Minimize your intake of sugary beverages, refined carbohydrates, and processed foods, as they can cause spikes in blood sugar levels. Opt for healthier alternatives such as water, herbal tea, whole grains, and fresh fruits.

- **Monitor Carbohydrate Intake:** Pay attention to the quantity and quality of carbohydrates in your diet, as they have the most significant impact on blood sugar levels. Choose complex carbohydrates that are high in fiber and have a lower glycemic index, such as whole grains, legumes, and non-starchy vegetables.

- **Control Portion Sizes:** Be mindful of portion sizes to avoid overeating and keep your blood sugar levels in check. Use measuring cups, spoons, or visual cues to help you estimate appropriate portion sizes, especially for carbohydrate-rich foods.

- **Eat Regularly:** Aim to eat balanced meals and snacks at regular intervals throughout the day to maintain steady blood sugar levels. Avoid skipping meals or going long periods without eating, as this can lead to fluctuations in blood sugar levels.

2. Exercise:

Physical activity is essential for diabetes management as it helps improve insulin sensitivity, lower blood sugar levels, and maintain a healthy weight. Here are some exercise recommendations:

- **Include Aerobic Exercise:** Engage in regular aerobic exercise such as walking, jogging, cycling, swimming, or dancing. Aim for at least 150 minutes of moderate-intensity aerobic activity per week, spread out over several days.

- **Incorporate Strength Training:** Include strength training exercises at least two days per week to build muscle mass and improve metabolic health. Use resistance bands, free weights, or bodyweight exercises to target major muscle groups.

- **Stay Active Throughout the Day:** Find opportunities to be active throughout the day, such as taking the stairs instead of the elevator, parking farther away from your destination, or doing household chores and gardening.

- **Monitor Blood Sugar Levels:** Check your blood sugar levels before and after exercise, especially if you're taking medication that can affect blood sugar levels. Adjust your food intake or medication as needed to prevent hypoglycemia during or after exercise.

3. Stress Management:

Chronic stress can contribute to insulin resistance and worsen blood sugar control in people with diabetes. Incorporating stress management techniques into your daily routine can help reduce stress levels and improve overall well-being. Here are some stress management strategies:

- **Practice Relaxation Techniques:** Incorporate relaxation techniques such as deep breathing exercises, meditation, yoga, or progressive muscle relaxation into your daily routine to help reduce stress and promote relaxation.

- **Stay Active:** Regular physical activity can help reduce stress levels and improve mood. Find activities that you enjoy and make them a regular part of your routine.

- **Prioritize Sleep:** Aim for 7-9 hours of quality sleep per night to support overall health and well-being. Establish a relaxing bedtime routine, create a comfortable sleep environment, and limit caffeine and screen time before bedtime.

- **Seek Support:** Reach out to friends, family members, or support groups for emotional support and encouragement. Talking to others who understand what you're going through can help alleviate feelings of stress and isolation.

Conclusion:

Incorporating healthy lifestyle changes such as a balanced diet, regular exercise, and stress management techniques is essential for long-term diabetes control. By making these changes, you can improve blood sugar levels, reduce the risk of complications, and enhance overall quality of life. Remember to work closely with your healthcare team to develop a personalized diabetes management plan that addresses your individual needs and preferences. With dedication and commitment to a healthy lifestyle, you can effectively manage diabetes and enjoy a full, active life.

CHAPTER NINE

Success Stories and Testimonials: Real People, Real Results

Success stories and testimonials from individuals who have experienced positive outcomes from using herbal remedies for diabetes management can provide inspiration and motivation for others on a similar journey. These real-life accounts offer insights into the effectiveness of herbal medicine and its impact on improving health and well-being. Let's explore some compelling success stories and testimonials from individuals who have benefited from incorporating herbal remedies into their diabetes management plans.

1. John's Journey to Better Blood Sugar Control:

John, a 55-year-old man with type 2 diabetes, struggled for years to manage his blood sugar levels despite conventional treatments. Frustrated with the side effects of medication and seeking alternative options, he decided to explore herbal remedies under the guidance of a qualified herbalist.

After incorporating bitter melon tea and fenugreek capsules into his daily routine, along with dietary changes and regular exercise, John noticed significant improvements in his blood sugar control. His A1C levels decreased, and he experienced fewer spikes and crashes throughout the day.

John's success story serves as a testament to the power of herbal medicine and lifestyle modifications in achieving better blood sugar control and overall health.

2. Sarah's Journey to Finding Balance with Gymnema Sylvestre:

Sarah, a 45-year-old woman with type 1 diabetes, struggled with sugar cravings and fluctuating blood sugar levels for years. Despite diligently managing her insulin regimen, she found it challenging to maintain stable blood sugar levels throughout the day.

Upon discovering gymnemasylvestre, also known as the "sugar destroyer," Sarah decided to give it a try. She incorporated gymnema tea into her daily routine and noticed a significant reduction in her sugar cravings and improved blood sugar control.

With the support of gymnemasylvestre and other lifestyle changes, such as mindful eating and stress management techniques, Sarah achieved greater balance in her blood sugar levels and experienced a renewed sense of well-being.

3. Mark's Journey to Overcoming Insulin Resistance with Cinnamon:

Mark, a 40-year-old man with prediabetes and insulin resistance, was determined to take control of his health and avoid progressing to type 2 diabetes. After researching natural remedies for insulin resistance, he learned about the potential benefits of cinnamon in improving insulin sensitivity.

Mark began incorporating cinnamon into his diet by adding it to his morning oatmeal and drinking cinnamon tea throughout the day. Over time, he noticed a gradual improvement in his insulin sensitivity and blood sugar levels.

With the support of cinnamon and other lifestyle modifications such as regular exercise and stress management, Mark successfully reversed his insulin resistance and achieved better blood sugar control.

Conclusion:

These success stories and testimonials from real people highlight the transformative power of herbal remedies in diabetes management. By incorporating herbal medicine into their daily routines, these individuals were able to achieve better blood sugar control, reduce reliance on medication, and improve their overall quality of life.

It's essential to approach herbal medicine with caution and consult with a qualified healthcare provider or herbalist before starting any new herbal regimen, especially if you have pre-existing health conditions or are taking medications. With proper guidance and personalized treatment plans, you too can experience the benefits of herbal remedies in managing diabetes and achieving optimal health and well-being.

BONUS: SOME HOLISTIC, HERBAL AND NATURAL MEASURES FOR HEEALTH AND WELLNESS

Manjakani:

Definition: Manjakani, also known as Quercus infectoria or oak gall, is a natural substance derived from the oak tree. It has been used for centuries in traditional medicine for its potential health benefits, particularly for women's health and vaginal tightening.

Ingredients: Manjakani contains various bioactive compounds, including tannins, flavonoids, and gallic acid. These compounds are believed to contribute to the herb's medicinal properties, including its potential as an astringent and antiseptic agent.

How to Prepare: Manjakani is typically available in powder, capsule, or liquid extract form. It can be taken orally or used topically depending on the intended use. For vaginal tightening, manjakani may be applied topically as a gel or inserted into the vagina in capsule form.

Dosage: The appropriate dosage of manjakani can vary depending on factors such as age, health status, and the specific preparation being used. It's important to follow the recommended dosage on the product label or consult with a qualified herbalist or healthcare professional for personalized guidance.

How to Use: Manjakani can be taken orally or used topically depending on the intended use. It's important to use manjakani products as directed and to discontinue use if any adverse effects occur.

Side Effects: Manjakani is generally considered safe for most people when used in moderate amounts. However, some individuals may experience allergic reactions or skin irritation when used topically. It's important to use manjakani under the guidance of a healthcare professional and to discontinue use if any adverse effects occur.

Red Clover:

Definition: Red clover, scientifically known as Trifolium pratense, is a flowering plant belonging to the legume family. It's native to Europe, Western Asia, and Northwest Africa but has been naturalized in many other regions. Red clover has been used in traditional medicine for various purposes, including its potential to support women's health and menopausal symptoms.

Ingredients: Red clover contains several bioactive compounds, including isoflavones (such as genistein and daidzein), flavonoids, and phytoestrogens. These compounds are believed to contribute to the herb's medicinal properties, including its potential as a hormone-balancing agent and its ability to support cardiovascular health.

How to Prepare: Red clover is typically prepared and consumed as an herbal tea or tincture. To make tea, dried red clover flowers are steeped in hot water for several minutes before being strained and consumed. Tinctures are prepared by steeping the flowers in alcohol or vinegar to extract their active compounds.

Dosage: The appropriate dosage of red clover can vary depending on factors such as age, health status, and the specific preparation being used. It's important to follow the recommended dosage on the product label or consult with a qualified herbalist or healthcare professional for personalized guidance.

How to Use: Red clover tea or tincture is typically taken orally. It's important to use red clover products as directed and to discontinue use if any adverse effects occur.

Side Effects: Red clover is generally considered safe for most people when used in moderate amounts. However, some individuals may experience allergic reactions or digestive upset. It may also interact with certain medications or have adverse effects in individuals with certain health conditions. It's important to use red clover under the guidance of a healthcare professional and to discontinue use if any adverse effects occur.

Red Raspberry:

Definition: Red raspberry, scientifically known as Rubus idaeus, is a species of raspberry native to Europe and northern Asia. It's widely cultivated for its delicious berries and has been used in traditional medicine for various purposes, including its potential to support women's health during pregnancy and childbirth.

Ingredients: Red raspberry contains several bioactive compounds, including flavonoids, ellagic acid, anthocyanins, and vitamin C. These compounds are believed to contribute to the herb's medicinal properties, including its potential as an antioxidant, anti-inflammatory, and uterine tonic.

How to Prepare: Red raspberry leaf is typically prepared and consumed as an herbal tea or infusion. To make tea, dried red raspberry leaves are steeped in hot water for several minutes before being strained and consumed.

Dosage: The appropriate dosage of red raspberry leaf can vary depending on factors such as age, health status, and the specific preparation being used. It's important to follow the recommended dosage on the product label or consult with a qualified herbalist or healthcare professional for personalized guidance.

How to Use: Red raspberry leaf tea is typically taken orally. It's often recommended for pregnant individuals in the later stages of pregnancy to support uterine health and prepare for childbirth.

It's important to use red raspberry leaf products as directed and to discontinue use if any adverse effects occur.

Side Effects: Red raspberry leaf is generally considered safe for most people when used in moderate amounts. However, some individuals may experience allergic reactions or digestive upset. Pregnant individuals should consult with a healthcare professional before using red raspberry leaf, especially if they have any underlying health conditions or are taking medications. It's important to use red raspberry leaf under the guidance of a healthcare professional and to discontinue use if any adverse effects occur.

Rhubarb:

Definition: Rhubarb, scientifically known as Rheum rhabarbarum, is a perennial plant cultivated for its edible stalks. While primarily used in culinary applications, rhubarb has also been utilized in traditional medicine for its potential health benefits, particularly for digestive health.

Ingredients: Rhubarb stalks contain various bioactive compounds, including anthraquinones (such as emodin and rhein), fiber, vitamins (such as vitamin K), and minerals (including calcium and potassium). These compounds are believed to contribute to the herb's medicinal properties, including its potential as a laxative and digestive aid.

How to Prepare: Rhubarb stalks are typically cooked before consumption, as the raw stalks are very tart and can be unpleasant to eat. They are often used in pies, crisps, jams, sauces, and other desserts, as well as in savory dishes. Rhubarb can also be used to make compotes, jams, and preserves.

Dosage: There is no specific dosage for rhubarb in culinary applications, as it is used as a food rather than a medicinal herb. However, when used for its potential laxative effects, it's important to consume rhubarb in moderation to avoid gastrointestinal upset.

How to Use: Rhubarb stalks can be chopped and cooked in various dishes, including pies, sauces, and jams. It's important to remove and discard the leaves, as they contain toxic compounds. When using rhubarb for its potential laxative effects, it's typically consumed as part of a cooked dish or in the form of a rhubarb-based herbal remedy.

Side Effects: Rhubarb stalks are generally safe for most people when consumed in moderate amounts as part of a balanced diet. However, excessive intake may lead to digestive upset or adverse effects due to the presence of oxalic acid, which can bind to calcium and form kidney stones in susceptible individuals. It's important to use rhubarb in moderation and to consult with a healthcare professional if you have any concerns or underlying health conditions.

Sarsaparilla:

Definition: Sarsaparilla refers to several species of plants belonging to the Smilax genus, including Smilax regelii and Smilax officinalis. It has been used historically in traditional medicine for its potential health benefits, particularly for its purported detoxifying and anti-inflammatory properties.

Ingredients: Sarsaparilla contains various bioactive compounds, including saponins (such as sarsaponin and smilagenin), flavonoids, phenolic acids, and sterols. These compounds are believed to contribute to the herb's medicinal properties, including its potential as a diuretic, blood purifier, and anti-inflammatory agent.

How to Prepare: Sarsaparilla root is typically prepared and consumed as an herbal tea, decoction, or tincture. To make tea, dried sarsaparilla root is steeped in hot water for several minutes before being strained and consumed. Decoctions involve boiling the root in water to extract its active compounds, while tinctures are prepared by steeping the root in alcohol or vinegar.

Dosage: The appropriate dosage of sarsaparilla can vary depending on factors such as age, health status, and the specific preparation being used. It's important to follow the recommended dosage on the product label or consult with a qualified herbalist or healthcare professional for personalized guidance.

How to Use: Sarsaparilla tea or tincture is typically taken orally. It's important to use sarsaparilla products as directed and to discontinue use if any adverse effects occur.

Side Effects: Sarsaparilla is generally considered safe for most people when used in moderate amounts. However, some individuals may experience allergic reactions or digestive upset. It may also interact with certain medications or have adverse effects in individuals with certain health conditions. It's important to use sarsaparilla under the guidance of a healthcare professional and to discontinue use if any adverse effects occur.

Tila:

Definition: Tila, also known as linden flower or lime blossom, refers to the flowers of the Tilia genus, primarily Tilia europaea and Tilia cordata. These trees are native to Europe, but they are also cultivated in other regions for their fragrant and medicinal flowers.

Ingredients: Tila flowers contain various bioactive compounds, including flavonoids, phenolic acids, and volatile oils. These compounds are believed to contribute to the herb's medicinal properties, including its potential as a mild sedative, anxiolytic, and anti-inflammatory agent.

How to Prepare: Tila flowers are typically prepared and consumed as an herbal tea or infusion. To make tea, dried tila flowers are steeped in hot water for several minutes before being strained and consumed.

Dosage: The appropriate dosage of tila can vary depending on factors such as age, health status, and the specific preparation being used. It's important to follow the recommended dosage on the product label or consult with a qualified herbalist or healthcare professional for personalized guidance.

How to Use: Tila tea is typically taken orally. It's often consumed in the evening as a calming bedtime beverage or during times of stress or anxiety. It's important to use tila products as directed and to discontinue use if any adverse effects occur.

Side Effects: Tila is generally considered safe for most people when used in moderate amounts. However, some individuals may experience allergic reactions or digestive upset. It may also interact with certain medications or have adverse effects in individuals with certain health conditions. It's important to use tila under the guidance of a healthcare professional and to discontinue use if any adverse effects occur.

Valerian:

Definition: Valerian, scientifically known as Valeriana officinalis, is a perennial flowering plant native to Europe and Asia. It has been used for centuries in traditional medicine for its potential calming and sedative effects.

Ingredients: Valerian root contains several bioactive compounds, including valerenic acid, valepotriates, and volatile oils. These compounds are believed to contribute to the herb's medicinal properties, including its potential as a sedative, anxiolytic, and sleep aid.

How to Prepare: Valerian root is typically prepared and consumed as an herbal tea, tincture, or capsule. To make tea, dried valerian root is steeped in hot water for several minutes before being strained and consumed. Tinctures are prepared by steeping the root in alcohol or vinegar to extract its active compounds.

Dosage: The appropriate dosage of valerian can vary depending on factors such as age, health status, and the specific preparation being used. It's important to follow the recommended dosage on the product label or consult with a qualified herbalist or healthcare professional for personalized guidance.

How to Use: Valerian tea, tincture, or capsules are typically taken orally. It's often consumed in the evening as a sleep aid or during times of stress or anxiety. It's important to use valerian products as directed and to discontinue use if any adverse effects occur.

Side Effects: Valerian is generally considered safe for most people when used in moderate amounts. However, some individuals may experience mild side effects such as drowsiness, headache, or gastrointestinal upset. It may also interact with certain medications or have adverse effects in individuals with certain health conditions. It's important to use valerian under the guidance of a healthcare professional and to discontinue use if any adverse effects occur.

Wild Cherry Bark:

Definition: Wild cherry bark, scientifically known as Prunus serotina, is the bark obtained from the black cherry tree native to North America. It has been used traditionally in Native American and folk medicine for its potential health benefits, particularly for respiratory and digestive issues.

Ingredients: Wild cherry bark contains various bioactive compounds, including cyanogenic glycosides (such as prunasin and amygdalin), flavonoids, and phenolic acids. These compounds are believed to contribute to the herb's medicinal properties, including its potential as an expectorant, cough suppressant, and mild sedative.

How to Prepare: Wild cherry bark is typically prepared and consumed as an herbal tea, decoction, or syrup. To make tea, dried wild cherry bark is steeped in hot water for several minutes before being strained and consumed. Decoctions involve boiling the bark in water to extract its active compounds, while syrups are made by simmering the bark with sugar or honey to create a thick, sweet liquid.

Dosage: The appropriate dosage of wild cherry bark can vary depending on factors such as age, health status, and the specific preparation being used. It's important to follow the recommended dosage on the product label or consult with a qualified herbalist or healthcare professional for personalized guidance.

How to Use: Wild cherry bark tea, decoction, or syrup is typically taken orally. It's often consumed to soothe coughs, sore throats, and other respiratory symptoms. It's important to use wild cherry bark products as directed and to discontinue use if any adverse effects occur.

Side Effects: Wild cherry bark is generally considered safe for most people when used in moderate amounts. However, it contains cyanogenic glycosides, which can release cyanide in the body when metabolized. While the risk of cyanide poisoning from consuming wild cherry bark is low when used appropriately, excessive intake or prolonged use may lead to adverse effects. It's important to use wild cherry bark under the guidance of a healthcare professional and to discontinue use if any adverse effects occur.

Yellowdock:

Definition: Yellowdock, scientifically known as Rumex crispus, is a perennial flowering plant native to Europe and western Asia but is also found in North America. It has a long history of use in traditional medicine, particularly among Indigenous peoples, for its potential health benefits.

Ingredients: Yellowdock root contains various bioactive compounds, including anthraquinone glycosides (such as emodin and chrysophanol), tannins, and vitamins (including vitamin A and vitamin C). These compounds are believed to contribute to the herb's medicinal properties, including its potential as a laxative, blood cleanser, and liver tonic.

How to Prepare: Yellowdock root is typically prepared and consumed as an herbal tea, tincture, or capsule. To make tea, dried yellowdock root is steeped in hot water for several minutes before being strained and consumed. Tinctures are prepared by steeping the root in alcohol or vinegar to extract its active compounds.

Dosage: The appropriate dosage of yellowdock can vary depending on factors such as age, health status, and the specific preparation being used. It's important to follow the recommended dosage on the product label or consult with a qualified herbalist or healthcare professional for personalized guidance.

How to Use: Yellowdock tea, tincture, or capsules are typically taken orally. It's often consumed to support digestion, promote bowel regularity, and cleanse the blood. It's important to use yellowdock products as directed and to discontinue use if any adverse effects occur.

Side Effects: Yellowdock is generally considered safe for most people when used in moderate amounts. However, some individuals may experience mild side effects such as gastrointestinal upset or allergic reactions. It may also interact with certain medications or have adverse effects in individuals with certain health conditions. It's important to use yellowdock under the guidance of a healthcare professional and to discontinue use if any adverse effects occur.

Yellowdock Root:

Definition: Yellowdock root, scientifically known as Rumex crispus, is the root of a perennial flowering plant native to Europe and western Asia, also found in North America. It has a long history of use in traditional medicine, particularly among Indigenous peoples, for its potential health benefits.

Ingredients: Yellowdock root contains various bioactive compounds, including anthraquinone glycosides (such as emodin and chrysophanol), tannins, and vitamins (including vitamin A and vitamin C). These compounds are believed to contribute to the herb's medicinal properties, including its potential as a laxative, blood cleanser, and liver tonic.

How to Prepare: Yellowdock root is typically prepared and consumed as an herbal tea, tincture, or capsule. To make tea, dried yellowdock root is steeped in hot water for several minutes before being strained and consumed. Tinctures are prepared by steeping the root in alcohol or vinegar to extract its active compounds.

Dosage: The appropriate dosage of yellowdock root can vary depending on factors such as age, health status, and the specific preparation being used. It's important to follow the recommended dosage on the product label or consult with a qualified herbalist or healthcare professional for personalized guidance.

How to Use: Yellowdock root tea, tincture, or capsules are typically taken orally. It's often consumed to support digestion, promote bowel regularity, and cleanse the blood. It's important to use yellowdock root products as directed and to discontinue use if any adverse effects occur.

Side Effects: Yellowdock root is generally considered safe for most people when used in moderate amounts. However, some individuals may experience mild side effects such as gastrointestinal upset or allergic reactions. It may also interact with certain medications or have adverse effects in individuals with certain health conditions. It's important to use yellowdock root under the guidance of a healthcare professional and to discontinue use if any adverse effects occur.

Agrimony:

Definition: Agrimony, scientifically known as Agrimonia eupatoria, is a perennial herbaceous plant native to Europe, Asia, and North America. It has a long history of use in traditional medicine, particularly in European folk medicine, for its potential health benefits.

Ingredients: Agrimony contains various bioactive compounds, including tannins, flavonoids, phenolic acids, and volatile oils. These compounds are believed to contribute to the herb's medicinal properties, including its potential as an astringent, anti-inflammatory, and digestive aid.

How to Prepare: Agrimony is typically prepared and consumed as an herbal tea, tincture, or poultice. To make tea, dried agrimony leaves and flowers are steeped in hot water for several minutes before being strained and consumed. Tinctures are prepared by steeping the herb in alcohol or vinegar to extract its active compounds.

Dosage: The appropriate dosage of agrimony can vary depending on factors such as age, health status, and the specific preparation being used. It's important to follow the recommended dosage on the product label or consult with a qualified herbalist or healthcare professional for personalized guidance.

How to Use: Agrimony tea, tincture, or poultice is typically taken orally or applied topically. It's often consumed to soothe gastrointestinal issues, such as indigestion and diarrhea, or used externally to treat skin conditions.

Side Effects: Agrimony is generally considered safe for most people when used in moderate amounts. However, some individuals may experience allergic reactions or gastrointestinal upset. It may also interact with certain medications or have adverse effects in individuals with certain health conditions. It's important to use agrimony under the guidance of a healthcare professional and to discontinue use if any adverse effects occur.

Alfalfa:

Definition: Alfalfa, scientifically known as Medicago sativa, is a flowering plant in the pea family native to Asia but cultivated worldwide. It's primarily grown as fodder for livestock, but it has also been used in traditional medicine for its potential health benefits.

Ingredients: Alfalfa contains various bioactive compounds, including vitamins (such as vitamin A, vitamin C, and vitamin K), minerals (including calcium, magnesium, and potassium), amino acids, and phytoestrogens. These compounds are believed to contribute to the herb's medicinal properties, including its potential as a nutritive tonic, diuretic, and hormone balancer.

How to Prepare: Alfalfa is typically consumed as sprouts, herbal tea, or in supplement form (such as capsules or tablets). To make tea, dried alfalfa leaves are steeped in hot water for several minutes before being strained and consumed.

Dosage: The appropriate dosage of alfalfa can vary depending on factors such as age, health status, and the specific preparation being used. It's important to follow the recommended dosage on the product label or consult with a qualified herbalist or healthcare professional for personalized guidance.

How to Use: Alfalfa sprouts, tea, or supplements are typically taken orally. It's often consumed as a dietary supplement to support overall health and well-being, as well as to promote kidney health and hormone balance.

Side Effects: Alfalfa is generally considered safe for most people when consumed in moderate amounts. However, some individuals may experience allergic reactions or digestive upset. It may also interact with certain medications or have adverse effects in individuals with certain health conditions, such as autoimmune diseases or hormone-sensitive conditions. Pregnant or breastfeeding individuals should consult with a healthcare professional before using alfalfa supplements. It's important to use alfalfa under the guidance of a healthcare professional and to discontinue use if any adverse effects occur.

Ashwagandha:

Definition: Ashwagandha, scientifically known as Withaniasomnifera, is a small shrub native to India, the Middle East, and parts of Africa. It has a long history of use in Ayurvedic medicine for its potential health benefits, particularly for its adaptogenic properties.

Ingredients: Ashwagandha root contains various bioactive compounds, including alkaloids (such as withanolides), steroidal lactones, and flavonoids. These compounds are believed to contribute to the herb's medicinal properties, including its potential as an adaptogen, anti-inflammatory, and immune-modulating agent.

How to Prepare: Ashwagandha is typically consumed as a powdered root, herbal tea, tincture, or in supplement form (such as capsules or tablets). To make tea, dried ashwagandha root is steeped in hot water for several minutes before being strained and consumed.

Dosage: The appropriate dosage of ashwagandha can vary depending on factors such as age, health status, and the specific preparation being used. It's important to follow the recommended dosage on the product label or consult with a qualified herbalist or healthcare professional for personalized guidance.

How to Use: Ashwagandha powder, tea, tincture, or supplements are typically taken orally. It's often consumed to support stress management, promote relaxation, and boost overall vitality and well-being.

Side Effects: Ashwagandha is generally considered safe for most people when used in moderate amounts. However, some individuals may experience mild side effects such as gastrointestinal upset or drowsiness. It may also interact with certain medications or have adverse effects in individuals with certain health conditions, such as autoimmune diseases or thyroid disorders. Pregnant or breastfeeding individuals should consult with a healthcare professional before using ashwagandha supplements. It's important to use ashwagandha under the guidance of a healthcare professional and to discontinue use if any adverse effects occur.

Astragalus:

Definition: Astragalus, scientifically known as Astragalus membranaceus, is a flowering plant native to China and Mongolia but also found in other parts of Asia. It has been used for centuries in traditional Chinese medicine for its potential health benefits, particularly for its immune-enhancing properties.

Ingredients: Astragalus root contains various bioactive compounds, including polysaccharides, saponins (such as astragalosides), flavonoids, and amino acids. These compounds are believed to contribute to the herb's medicinal properties, including its potential as an adaptogen, immunomodulator, and anti-inflammatory agent.

How to Prepare: Astragalus is typically consumed as a powdered root, herbal tea, tincture, or in supplement form (such as capsules or tablets). To make tea, dried astragalus root slices are simmered in water for several minutes before being strained and consumed.

Dosage: The appropriate dosage of astragalus can vary depending on factors such as age, health status, and the specific preparation being used. It's important to follow the recommended dosage on the product label or consult with a qualified herbalist or healthcare professional for personalized guidance.

How to Use: Astragalus powder, tea, tincture, or supplements are typically taken orally. It's often consumed to support immune function, promote vitality, and enhance overall well-being.

Side Effects: Astragalus is generally considered safe for most people when used in moderate amounts. However, some individuals may experience mild side effects such as gastrointestinal upset or allergic reactions. It may also interact with certain medications or have adverse effects in individuals with certain health conditions, such as autoimmune diseases or diabetes. Pregnant or breastfeeding individuals should consult with a healthcare professional before using astragalus supplements. It's important to use astragalus under the guidance of a healthcare professional and to discontinue use if any adverse effects occur.

Black Cohosh:

Definition: Black cohosh, scientifically known as Actaea racemosa (formerly Cimicifuga racemosa), is a perennial herb native to North America. It has a long history of use in traditional Native American medicine and later in folk medicine for its potential health benefits, particularly for women's health.

Ingredients: Black cohosh root contains various bioactive compounds, including triterpene glycosides (such as actein and cimicifugoside), phenolic acids, and flavonoids. These compounds are believed to contribute to the herb's medicinal properties, including its potential as a hormone-balancing agent and its ability to relieve menopausal symptoms.

How to Prepare: Black cohosh is typically consumed as a powdered root, herbal tea, tincture, or in supplement form (such as capsules or tablets). To make tea, dried black cohosh root is steeped in hot water for several minutes before being strained and consumed.

Dosage: The appropriate dosage of black cohosh can vary depending on factors such as age, health status, and the specific preparation being used. It's important to follow the recommended dosage on the product label or consult with a qualified herbalist or healthcare professional for personalized guidance.

How to Use: Black cohosh powder, tea, tincture, or supplements are typically taken orally. It's often used by women to support hormonal balance, relieve menopausal symptoms such as hot flashes and night sweats, and promote overall well-being.

Side Effects: Black cohosh is generally considered safe for most people when used in moderate amounts. However, some individuals may experience mild side effects such as gastrointestinal upset or allergic reactions. It may also interact with certain medications or have adverse effects in individuals with certain health conditions, such as liver disease or hormone-sensitive conditions. Pregnant or breastfeeding individuals should consult with a healthcare professional before using black cohosh supplements. It's important to use black cohosh under the guidance of a healthcare professional and to discontinue use if any adverse effects occur.

Blessed Thistle:

Definition: Blessed thistle, scientifically known as Cnicusbenedictus, is an annual or biennial herb native to the

Mediterranean region but also found in other parts of Europe, Asia, and North Africa. It has been used historically in traditional medicine for its potential health benefits, particularly for digestive and liver health.

Ingredients: Blessed thistle contains various bioactive compounds, including sesquiterpene lactones (such as cnicin), flavonoids, tannins, and essential oils. These compounds are believed to contribute to the herb's medicinal properties, including its potential as a digestive tonic, appetite stimulant, and liver tonic.

How to Prepare: Blessed thistle is typically consumed as an herbal tea, tincture, or in supplement form (such as capsules or tablets). To make tea, dried blessed thistle leaves and flowers are steeped in hot water for several minutes before being strained and consumed.

Dosage: The appropriate dosage of blessed thistle can vary depending on factors such as age, health status, and the specific preparation being used. It's important to follow the recommended dosage on the product label or consult with a qualified herbalist or healthcare professional for personalized guidance.

How to Use: Blessed thistle tea, tincture, or supplements are typically taken orally. It's often used to support digestion, stimulate appetite, and promote liver health.

Side Effects: Blessed thistle is generally considered safe for most people when used in moderate amounts. However, some individuals may experience mild side effects such as gastrointestinal upset or allergic reactions. It may also interact with certain medications or have adverse effects in individuals with certain health conditions, such as hormone-sensitive conditions or bleeding disorders. Pregnant or breastfeeding individuals should consult with a healthcare professional before using blessed thistle supplements. It's important to use blessed thistle under the guidance of a healthcare professional and to discontinue use if any adverse effects occur.

Cat's Claw:

Definition: Cat's claw, scientifically known as Uncaria tomentosa, is a woody vine native to the Amazon rainforest and other parts of Central and South America. It has been used for centuries in traditional medicine by indigenous peoples for its potential health benefits.

Ingredients: Cat's claw contains various bioactive compounds, including alkaloids (such as oxindole alkaloids and quinovic acid glycosides), polyphenols, and other phytochemicals. These compounds are believed to contribute to the herb's medicinal properties, including its potential as an immune enhancer, anti-inflammatory, and antioxidant.

How to Prepare: Cat's claw is typically consumed as an herbal tea, tincture, or in supplement form (such as capsules or tablets). To make tea, dried cat's claw bark or leaves are steeped in hot water for several minutes before being strained and consumed.

Dosage: The appropriate dosage of cat's claw can vary depending on factors such as age, health status, and the specific preparation being used. It's important to follow the recommended dosage on the product label or consult with a qualified herbalist or healthcare professional for personalized guidance.

How to Use: Cat's claw tea, tincture, or supplements are typically taken orally. It's often used to support immune function, reduce inflammation, and promote overall well-being.

Side Effects: Cat's claw is generally considered safe for most people when used in moderate amounts. However, some individuals may experience mild side effects such as gastrointestinal upset or allergic reactions. It may also interact with certain medications or have adverse effects in individuals with certain health conditions, such as autoimmune diseases or bleeding disorders. Pregnant or breastfeeding individuals should consult with a healthcare professional before using cat's claw supplements. It's important to use cat's claw under the guidance of a healthcare professional and to discontinue use if any adverse effects occur.

Cleavers:

Definition: Cleavers, scientifically known as Galium aparine, is a herbaceous annual plant native to Europe, North America, Asia, and Australia. It has a long history of use in traditional medicine for its potential health benefits.

Ingredients: Cleavers contains various bioactive compounds, including iridoid glycosides, flavonoids, tannins, and mucilage. These compounds are believed to contribute to the herb's medicinal properties, including its potential as a diuretic, lymphatic tonic, and mild astringent.

How to Prepare: Cleavers is typically consumed as an herbal tea, infusion, or in fresh salads. To make tea, dried cleavers leaves and stems are steeped in hot water for several minutes before being strained and consumed. It can also be used topically as a poultice or infused oil for skin conditions.

Dosage: The appropriate dosage of cleavers can vary depending on factors such as age, health status, and the specific preparation being used. It's important to follow the recommended dosage on the product label or consult with a qualified herbalist or healthcare professional for personalized guidance.

How to Use: Cleavers tea, infusion, or fresh leaves are typically taken orally. It's often used to support lymphatic drainage, promote urinary tract health, and soothe inflammation. Topically, cleavers can be applied to the skin to alleviate itching, irritation, or minor wounds.

Side Effects: Cleavers is generally considered safe for most people when consumed in moderate amounts. However, some individuals may experience allergic reactions or gastrointestinal upset. It may also interact with certain medications or have adverse effects in individuals with certain health conditions. Pregnant or breastfeeding individuals should consult with a healthcare professional before using cleavers supplements. It's important to use cleavers under the guidance of a healthcare professional and to discontinue use if any adverse effects occur.

Eucalyptus:

Definition: Eucalyptus refers to a genus of flowering trees and shrubs, primarily native to Australia but also found in other parts of the world. Eucalyptus essential oil, extracted from the leaves of certain species, has a long history of use in traditional medicine for its potential health benefits.

Ingredients: Eucalyptus essential oil contains various bioactive compounds, including eucalyptol (cineole), terpenes, and flavonoids. These compounds are believed to contribute to the oil's medicinal properties, including its potential as an expectorant, decongestant, antiseptic, and anti-inflammatory.

How to Prepare: Eucalyptus essential oil can be used in aromatherapy, diffused in the air, or diluted and applied topically to the skin. It can also be added to steam inhalations or chest rubs to help relieve respiratory symptoms.

Dosage: The appropriate dosage of eucalyptus essential oil can vary depending on factors such as age, health status, and the specific application being used. It's important to follow the recommended dosage on the product label or consult with a qualified aromatherapist or healthcare professional for personalized guidance.

How to Use: Eucalyptus essential oil can be used aromatically, topically, or internally, depending on the intended application. It's often used to alleviate respiratory congestion, soothe sore muscles, promote relaxation, and support overall well-being.

Side Effects: Eucalyptus essential oil is generally considered safe for most people when used appropriately. However, it can be toxic if ingested in large amounts and should not be applied directly to the skin without proper dilution. Some individuals may experience allergic reactions or respiratory irritation when exposed to eucalyptus oil. It's important to use eucalyptus oil with caution, especially around children and pets. Pregnant or breastfeeding individuals should consult with a healthcare professional before using eucalyptus oil. If any adverse effects occur, discontinue use and seek medical attention.

Feverfew:

Definition: Feverfew, scientifically known as Tanacetum parthenium, is a perennial herb native to Europe but also found in other parts of the world. It has a long history of use in traditional medicine, particularly in European folk medicine, for its potential health benefits.

Ingredients: Feverfew contains various bioactive compounds, including sesquiterpene lactones (such as parthenolide), flavonoids, and volatile oils. These compounds are believed to contribute to the herb's medicinal properties, including its potential as an anti-inflammatory, analgesic, and migraine prophylactic.

How to Prepare: Feverfew is typically consumed as an herbal tea, tincture, or in supplement form (such as capsules or tablets). To make tea, dried feverfew leaves and flowers are steeped in hot water for several minutes before being strained and consumed.

Dosage: The appropriate dosage of feverfew can vary depending on factors such as age, health status, and the specific preparation being used. It's important to follow the recommended dosage on the product label or consult with a qualified herbalist or healthcare professional for personalized guidance.

How to Use: Feverfew tea, tincture, or supplements are typically taken orally. It's often used to alleviate headaches, including migraines, and to support overall well-being.

Side Effects: Feverfew is generally considered safe for most people when used in moderate amounts. However, some individuals may experience mild side effects such as gastrointestinal upset or allergic reactions. It may also interact with certain medications or have adverse effects in individuals with certain health conditions, such as bleeding disorders or pregnancy. It's important to use feverfew under the guidance of a healthcare professional and to discontinue use if any adverse effects occur.

Ginseng:

Definition: Ginseng refers to several species of perennial plants belonging to the Panax genus, including Panax ginseng (Asian ginseng) and Panax quinquefolius (American ginseng). Ginseng has been used for centuries in traditional medicine, particularly in East Asia, for its potential health benefits.

Ingredients: Ginseng root contains various bioactive compounds, including ginsenosides, polysaccharides, and peptides. These compounds are believed to contribute to the herb's medicinal properties, including its potential as an adaptogen, immune enhancer, and cognitive booster.

How to Prepare: Ginseng is typically consumed as a powdered root, herbal tea, tincture, or in supplement form (such as capsules or tablets). To make tea, dried ginseng root slices are simmered in water for several minutes before being strained and consumed.

Dosage: The appropriate dosage of ginseng can vary depending on factors such as age, health status, and the specific preparation being used. It's important to follow the recommended dosage on the product label or consult with a qualified herbalist or healthcare professional for personalized guidance.

How to Use: Ginseng powder, tea, tincture, or supplements are typically taken orally. It's often used to support energy levels, enhance cognitive function, and promote overall well-being.

Side Effects: Ginseng is generally considered safe for most people when used in moderate amounts. However, some individuals may experience mild side effects such as insomnia, gastrointestinal upset, or headaches. It may also interact with certain medications or have adverse effects in individuals with certain health conditions, such as high blood pressure or diabetes. Pregnant or breastfeeding individuals should consult with a healthcare professional before using ginseng supplements. It's important to use ginseng under the guidance of a healthcare professional and to discontinue use if any adverse effects occur.

Chickweed:

Definition: Chickweed, scientifically known as Stellaria media, is an annual herbaceous plant native to Europe but naturalized in many other parts of the world. It's often considered a common weed but has been used historically in traditional medicine for its potential health benefits.

Ingredients: Chickweed contains various bioactive compounds, including flavonoids, saponins, mucilage, and vitamins (such as vitamin C). These compounds are believed to contribute to the herb's medicinal properties, including its potential as a demulcent, anti-inflammatory, and mild diuretic.

How to Prepare: Chickweed is typically consumed as an herbal tea, infusion, or in fresh salads. To make tea, dried chickweed leaves and flowers are steeped in hot water for several minutes before being strained and consumed. It can also be used topically as a poultice or infused oil for skin conditions.

Dosage: The appropriate dosage of chickweed can vary depending on factors such as age, health status, and the specific preparation being used. It's important to follow the recommended dosage on the product label or consult with a qualified herbalist or healthcare professional for personalized guidance.

How to Use: Chickweed tea, infusion, or fresh leaves are typically taken orally. It's often used to soothe inflammation, support digestion, and promote overall well-being. Topically, chickweed can be applied to the skin to alleviate itching, irritation, or minor wounds.

Side Effects: Chickweed is generally considered safe for most people when consumed in moderate amounts. However, some individuals may experience allergic reactions or gastrointestinal upset. It may also interact with certain medications or have adverse effects in individuals with certain health conditions. Pregnant or breastfeeding individuals should consult with a healthcare professional before using chickweed supplements. It's important to use chickweed under the guidance of a healthcare professional and to discontinue use if any adverse effects occur.

THE END